Learning is the Fountain of Youth.
No matter how old you are,
You mustn't stop growing.

--Deng Ming-Dao

Fantastic Feet!
Exercises to Strengthen the Ankles, Arches & Toes
ISBN 10: 0-9771576-0-1
ISBN 13: 978-0-9771570-0-0
Copyright © MMV by Aliesa R. George
P.O. Box 3526
Wichita, KS 67201-3526 USA

Published by Centerworks® Pilates Institute
P.O. Box 3526 ▪ Wichita, KS 67201-3526 USA
www.CenterworksPilates.com

Printed in the United States of America
All rights reserved under International Copyright Law.
Contents and/or cover may not be reproduced in whole or in part in any form without the expressed written consent of the publisher.

———————— Note from the Author ————————

Our feet are the most used and abused part of the body.

The arches of the feet provide us with flexibility, help to absorb shock, distribute the weight of the body, and assist the feet in adapting to surface changes when walking, running, & climbing.

Lack of proper foot/arch strength & flexibility can contribute to fallen arches, ankle, knee, hip, back, shoulder, and neck problems. Improving our posture really does start from the ground up!

In college I was given orthodics to wear in my shoes. (I've always had very flat feet, and a bad lower back.) This new support was a shock to my system, I noticed new pains in my knees, hips, and back as a result of a more lifted arch and proper body alignment. It took time, and the help of a very good osteopathic physician, for my muscles and joints to adjust to new alignment and improved posture that the orthodics provided.

While I vigorously exercised every other part of my body, I had never been taught corrective exercises for my feet. In fact, I don't think it even crossed my mind that if I knew the right things to do I could strengthen my feet and use my own muscles to lift my arches! It wasn't until I started learning Pilates that the importance of the feet became evident. Then I began to see how muscle imbalances in other parts of my body related back to my feet. When I first began practicing some of these exercises it became clear how uncoordinated and weak my feet and lower legs really were. On the bright side, with practice the exercises got easier, muscles stronger, and along the way other aches and pains began to diminish.

I have taught the exercises in this book to many clients and teachers. They make great homework assignments! Whether you incorporate just a few exercises into your regular workout program, or do an entire foot fitness session, great results can be achieved. Many clients have seen wonderful improvement by practicing this simple series of exercises. Change doesn't happen overnight, but with patience and persistance you can gain mastery over your toes, enjoy good health, and have fantastic feet!

Special Thanks

I would like to express my thanks to all the wonderful Dance and Pilates teachers I have had who have shared their knowledge with me and inspired me to continue learning.

The exercises in this book come from a variety of sources and years of experience. I am sure that as I attempt to credit everyone I will forget to mention an important mentor, so advance apologies for the foot in my mouth if I've left anybody out.

Those responsible for my inspiration and education include: Stan & Sharon Rogers, all the faculty at the TCU Dance Department, David Mooney, Romana Kryzanowska, Sari Pace, Michele Larson, Coleen Glenn, and especially Dianne Miller.

I would also like to express my appreciation to the Pilates Method Alliance for making it possible to learn from the First Generation Pilates teachers: Mary Bowen, Ron Fletcher, Cathy Grant and Lolita San Miguel.

The gifts that these teachers have to impart is so very special. I have been blessed to enjoy insight and education from them all.

Table of Contents

Special Thanks 5

Safety Precautions 9

The Benefit of Exercising the Feet 11

Seated Footwork 19

      L-Sit Exercises 22

      Hook-Sit Exercises 34

      Chair Exercises 40

Terrific Toe Series 47

Theraband Foot Series 57

Standing Footwork Series 65

Quick Reference 77

Foot Reflexology and Massage 79

About the Author 83

References 84

Recommended Resources 85

Safety Precautions

The following series of foot exercises can assist you in the development of improved strength & flexibility for your toes, arches, feet, and lower legs.

Before following any advice, it is recommended that you consult with your physician if you suffer from any health problems or special conditions, or are in doubt about the suitability of any exercise.

Please Note:
Practicing foot exercises can be sneaky. You may not feel like you're doing much work, while you are exercising. I always notice that I've worked my feet the day after I've done my Fantastic Feet workout.

- Start with just a few repetitions 3-5, and only a few exercises.
- Pay attention to how your feet feel the next day.
- Adjust your workouts from there, gradually increasing the number of exercises and challenge.

The Benefit of Exercising the Feet

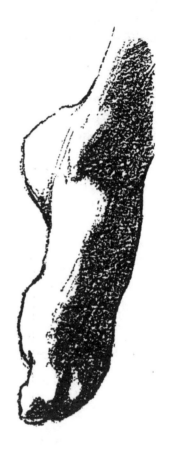

- Footwork exercises are beneficial for everyone, but can be especially helpful if you have flat feet, ankle inversion/eversion, bunions, or need to improve leg alignment.

- The following exercises may be challenging if you have any of the above mentioned problems. Hang in there, they will get easier quickly as the muscles in the feet/arches become stronger and more supple.

- Use your hands as much as needed to assist when learning the exercises. Eventually, the feet should do all the work.

- Footwork exercises are great homework.

- Remember, good posture begins from the ground up!

The Important Role of the Feet for Movement & Health

Our feet support the whole body. They provide levers that push the body off the ground while walking and running. They form a resilient and springy base that accepts the weight of the body on both flat & uneven surfaces, while giving us a wider base of support for balance when standing. The muscles of the arch help to absorb shock as we move. Think of the ankles and toes like the flippers in a pin ball machine. They push to propel, our body forward to walk, run, hop, skip, and jump.

Framework of the Foot

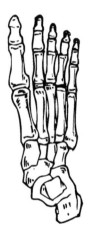

14 phalanges (toes)

5 metatarsal (sole)

7 tarsal bones (ankle)

26 BONES

Arches of the Feet

Two longitudinal arches — lengthwise from the heel to the ball of the foot.
    1 ~ Medial (inner) — from heel to 1st three toes
    2 ~ Lateral (outer) — from heel to last 2 toes

Two transverse metatarsal arches — across the width of the foot.
    3 ~ Posterior — base of the metatarsal bones
    4 ~ Anterior — distal/heads of metatarsals

(See diagram on the following page.)

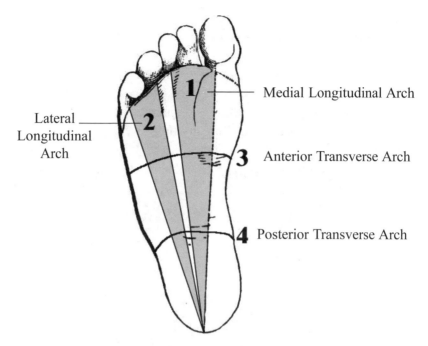

Muscles of the Foot and Lower Leg

Weak or imbalanced muscles can pull the bones out of place resulting in a variety of foot ailments. Over time these problems can lead to injuries of the knee, hip, spine, and other body systems that have been affected by poor posture habits.

All of the muscles listed below play an important role in proper strength & support of the ankles and arches.

<u>Intrinsic Muscles of the Foot</u>
Abductor hallucis
Flexor digitorum brevis
Abductor digiti minimi
Quadratus plantae
Lumbricals
Flexor hallucis brevis
Adductor hallucis
Flexor digiti minimi brevis
Dorsal interossei
Plantar interossei
Extensor digitorum brevis
Extensor hallucis brevis

<u>Muscles of the Leg & Foot</u>
Tibialis anterior
Extensor digitorum longus
Extensor hallucis longus
Peroneus tertuis
Peroneus longus
Peroneus brevis
Gastrocnemius
Soleus
Plantaris
Flexor digitorum longus
Flexor hallucis longus
Tibialis posterior

The Benefit of Exercising the Feet

Standing Foot Placement

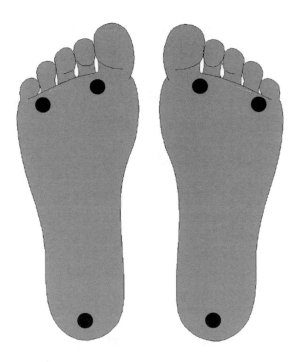

Awareness for Improving Posture Habits

Weight should be on the ball of the foot with equal weight on the big toe, little toe & center of the heel, evenly distributed like a tripod. Arches of the feet should be lifted. While the toes muscles will be active to help lift the arches, the toes should not curl under, but instead spread, lengthen and reach away from the heel.

- ☑ Notice if the weight is more on the heels.
- ☑ Notice if the weight is more to the big toes, rolled inward.
- ☑ Notice if the weight is more to the little toes, rolled outward.

It is not unusual for weight bearing on the feet to be different on the right & left legs.

Improving Your Foot Placement

It is very difficult to change habits while you are in a standing position. When weight-bearing the knees take additional stress when re-adjusting the feet. The exercises in this book that are seated and lying down are the best ones to begin with and are excellent for a home workout program.

If you'd like additional assistance with correcting muscle imbalance and safely changing your habits. Find a qualified Pilates teacher/studio in your area. By utilizing the Pilates Reformer, Cadillac Matwork, Chairs & Supplemental Equipment, the correct muscles can be strengthened & stretched without undue stress on the joints. With Pilates, good posture is practiced in a non-weight bearing position first, strengthening new muscles to assist in supporting the body. New habits can then be transferred back to everyday life activities.

For additional information on improving standing and seated posture refer to the workbook and video, *Posture Principles for Health* **also written by Aliesa R. George.**
(see pg. 90)

Movement of the Foot

For the exercises in this book flexion of the foot/ankle means dorsiflexion, pointing the foot describes plantar flexion.

The second toe is the reference on the foot for adduction & abduction of the toes. (Toes spreading apart and squeezing together.)

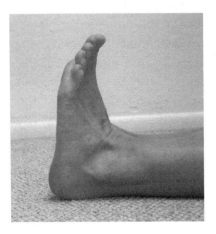

Dorsiflexion: Movement of the top of foot towards the shin bone. "Flex."

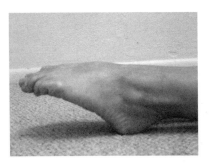

Plantar flexion: Movement of the sole of the foot downward toward the floor. "Point."

Fantastic Feet!

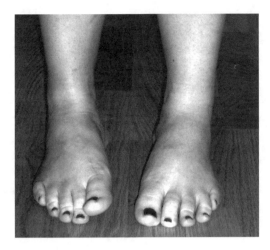

Inversion: Turning the sole of the foot inward.

Weight on the outer edge of the foot-soles of the feet face towards each other. (Prone to sprained ankles.)

This position may also be referred to as supination.

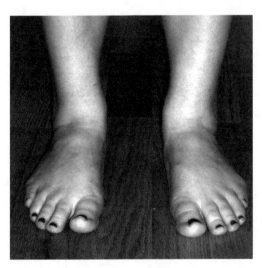

Eversion: Turning the sole of the foot outward.

Weight on the inner edge of the foot-soles of the feet face away from each other. "Fallen arches" or "flat feet."

May also be referred to as pronation.

Fantastic Feet!
Seated Footwork Exercises

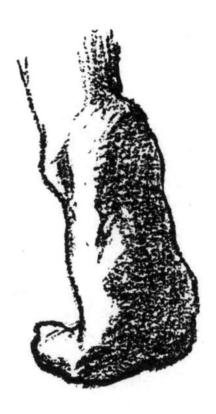

Seated Footwork Exercises

For All Seated Exercises

- Keep the feet and knees pointed straight ahead.
- Ankles should not roll in or out.
- Weight evenly distributed between the big and little toe.
- Heels stay hidden behind the rest of the feet when on your tippy toes.
- Be sure you are working evenly through both feet.
- Bending over to look at your feet will not help improve your posture.

It can be helpful to watch your ankle alignment while executing these exercises. Sit in front of a mirror, so you can sit tall and still watch your leg and foot alignment.

Please note: If it is difficult for you to get up and down from the floor, all of the L-Sit, Hook-Sit, and toe series exercises can be done in a chair.

Maintaining Good Alignment

Regardless of the exercise and your body position (L-Sit, Hook-Sit, Hook-Lying, Seated, or Standing) it is very important to maintain good alignment.

- The knee should be in line with the hip and centered over the foot.
- The ankle should be centered between the big and little toes (not rolled in or out.)
- The toes should be pointed straight ahead.

Here are some examples of good, and not so good, foot and leg placement.

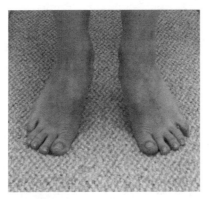

Bad Placement — Ankles Rolled In

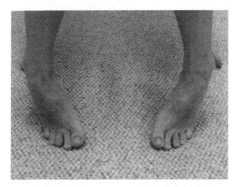

Bad Placement — Ankles Rolled Out

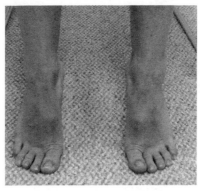

Good Ankle Alignment

L-Sit Exercises

L-Sit Position

- For the L-Sit exercises posture should be tall & vertical—ears over shoulders, shoulders over hips.

- Legs are together and extend forward at a 90 degree angle.

- If your leg muscles are not very flexible to help maintain a good position, sit on a phone book or firm pillow to help stack the spine and reduce the stretch on the back of the legs.

- If you need additional back support, sit against a wall.

- This series can also be done lying down.

Fantastic Feet!

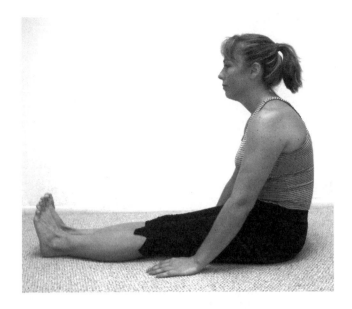

L-Sit: Bad Posture

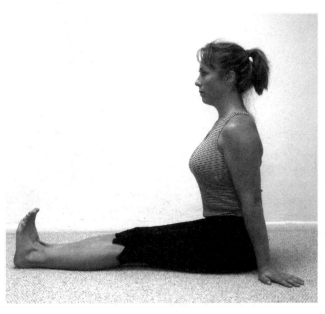

L-Sit: Good Posture

Seated Footwork Exercises

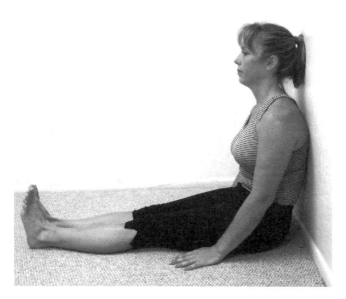

Bad Posture: L-Sit Against Wall

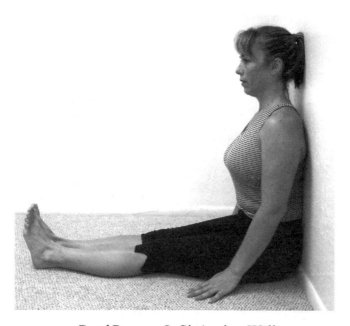

Good Posture: L-Sit Against Wall

Fantastic Feet!

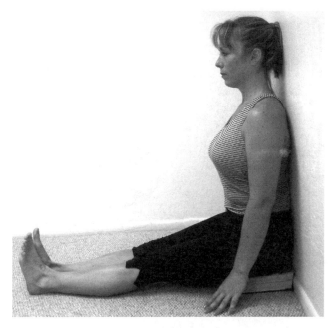

Modified L-Sit Against Wall with Book
(for back support)

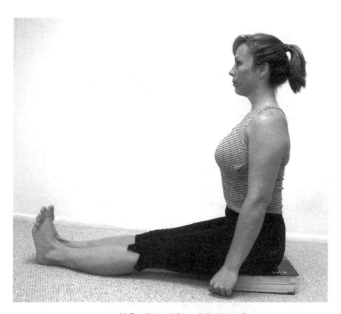

Modified L-Sit with Book
(for tight hamstrings)

Seated Footwork Exercises

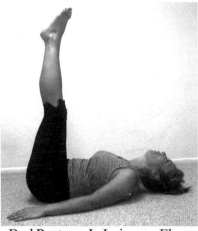

Bad Posture: L-Lying on Floor

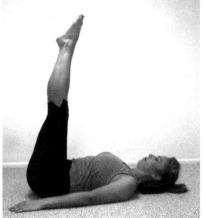

Good Posture: L-Lying on Floor with Pillow for Neck Support

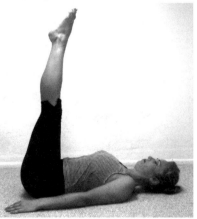

Good Posture: L-Lying on Floor

L-Sit Exercise Series

Sole Searching - part one

- Keep the legs straight and together throughout the exercise.
- Begin with flexed feet.
- Turn at the ankle so that the soles of the feet come together.
- Rotate the ankles back to the start position.
- Repeat 5-10x

When starting it may be difficult to keep the legs still and just turn the ankles and the feet. Don't worry if the soles don't make it all the way together, go as far as you can without changing the position of the legs.

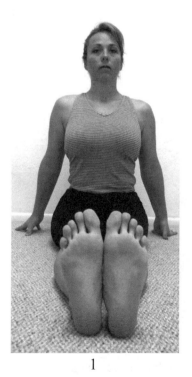

1

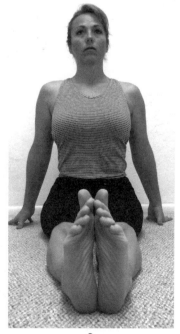

2

L-Sit Exercise Series

Sole Searching - part two

Once the soles are together, point and flex the feet 3 times while continuing to rotate the ankles to get more of the soles touching. Finish with the feet flexed and ankles back to parallel (your starting position.) 3x3

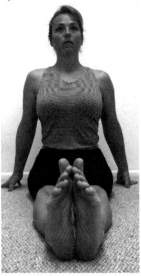

Soles together

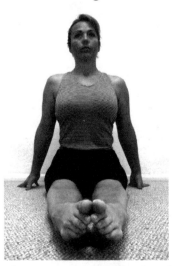

Soles together — point and flex feet three times

Fantastic Feet!

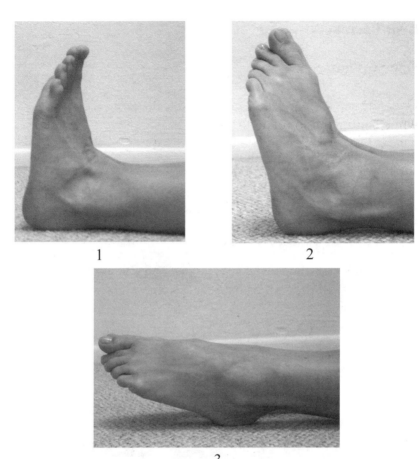

Repeat 2 & 3 with the soles together. Repeat 3 times.

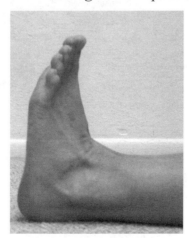

Finish position

Seated Footwork Exercises

L-Sit Exercises

Point & Flex - 5x

- Begin in a good L-Sit position, feet flexed.

- Point the ankles, then use the muscles under the foot to lengthen and point the toes.

- Continue to move the ankle and toes closer to the floor by actively contracting the bottom of the foot.

- Flex the toes back first, then flex the ankle.

- Movement should be very precise and articulate. heel/ball/toes—toes/ball/heel. Repeat this exercise 5 times.

1

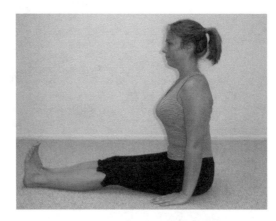

2

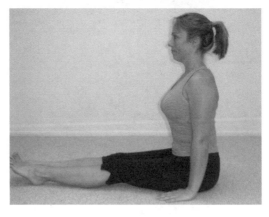

Fantastic Feet!

3

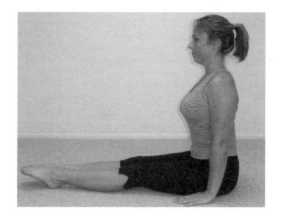

4

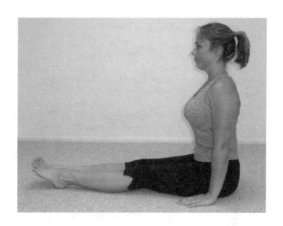

5

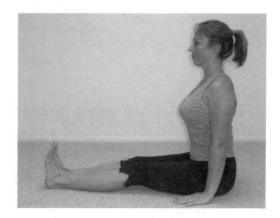

Seated Footwork Exercises

L-Sit Exercises

Toe Curl Combo - 5x. Curl toes/point & flex.

- Begin in a good L-Sit position, feet flexed.
- Keeping the ankles flexed, curl the toes and release 3x.
- Then do one repetition of the Point & Flex exercise.
- Repeat the combination 3 Toe Curls/1 Point & Flex.- 5 times.

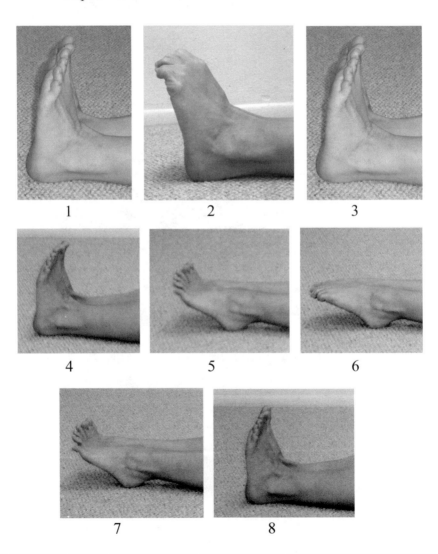

Fantastic Feet!

L-Sit Exercises

Ankle Circles - 3-5x. Both directions.

- Begin in a good L-Sit position, feet flexed.
- Keep the thighs still and knees pointing straight to the ceiling.
- Draw a large circle with both feet moving in the same direction.
- Move both feet to the right, point the toes to the floor, move the feet to the left, and finish with feet flexed.
- 3-5 repetitions.

Options: Alternate the circles—right/left. Do 3-5 circles starting to the right, then 3-5 circles left.

1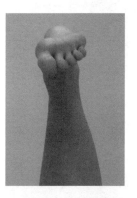

3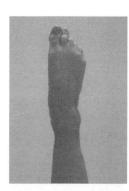

2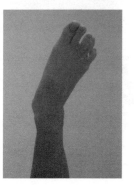

4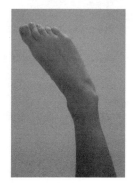

Seated Footwork Exercises

Hook-Sit Exercises

Hook-Sit Positions

From your L-Sit position, reach the arms overhead, and circle them around to the back to support on the hands. Hinge the body back on a diagonal. You may need to adjust the arms back farther. Keeping a tall-lifted body position, use the abdominals to draw the knees towards the chest until the feet are flat on the floor.

Watch that the shoulders stay away from the ears, no slouching, elbows remain soft. If supporting on your arms is too much for your wrists, rest on you elbows.

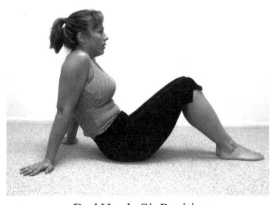

Bad Hook-Sit Position

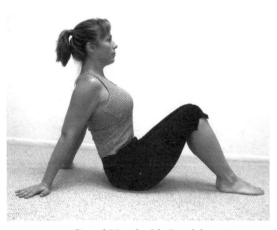

Good Hook-Sit Position

Hook-Sit

Toe Presses - 3x3

- Begin in a good Hook-Sit position, feet flat.

- Lift the heels rising to the balls of the feet. Be sure to keep the ankles in good alignment.

- Keeping the heels lifted, push through the toes to point the feet.

- With the heels still up, break at the toes to roll back down to the balls of the feet. Repeat this push to point and release 3 times before setting the heels down.

This exercise can be a real foot cramper! Actively use the muscles on the soles of the feet to point the toes. Try not to curl the toes under, but push through the toe bones—keeping the toes stretched long.

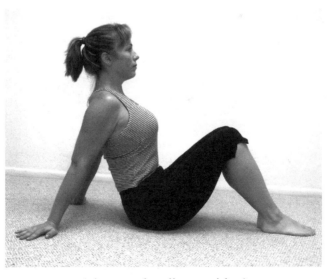

1 (start and ending position)

Hook-Sit: Toe Presses

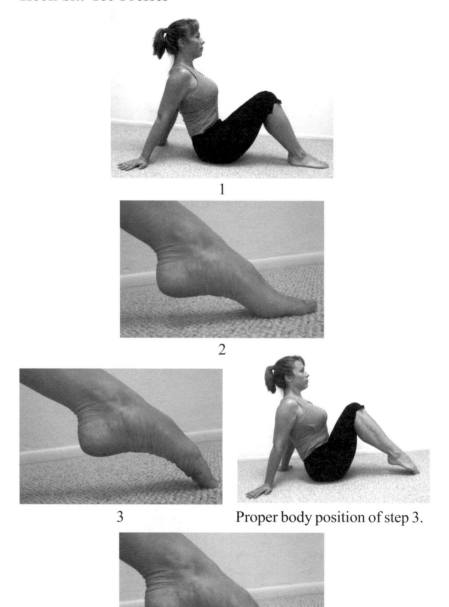

Proper body position of step 3.

Do positions 2-4, three times and then end with position 1.

Hook-Sit

Ankle Hinge - 5x. Flex ankles w/toes relaxed.

- Begin with the feet flat on the floor.
- Without flexing the toe joints, hinge at the ankle to flex the foot.
- Release to set the foot down.
- Repeat 5 times.

a. *optional/add Toe Curls 3x3*
   While the ankle is flexed, curl the toes & release 3 times before setting the foot down.

b. *optional/Taps 20-30x*
   At a brisk tempo, tap the foot, hinging from the ankle.

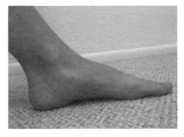
1

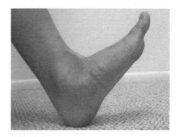
2

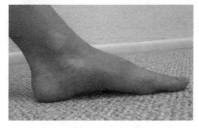
3

Recommended Exercise: After performing the Hook-Sit series, lie on your back and repeat Ankle circles. (pg. 33)

Seated Footwork Exercises

Hook-Sit

Flex & Point 3-5x

- Begin in a good Hook-Sit position, feet flat.

- Lift the heels rising to the balls of the feet. Be sure to keep the ankles in good alignment.

- Keeping the heels lifted, push through the toes to point the feet.

- With the heels still up, break at the toes to roll back down to the balls of the feet.

- Set the heels down.

- Flex the toes back, then flex the ankles.

- Roll back to the starting position by placing the ball of the foot on the floor first, then the toes.

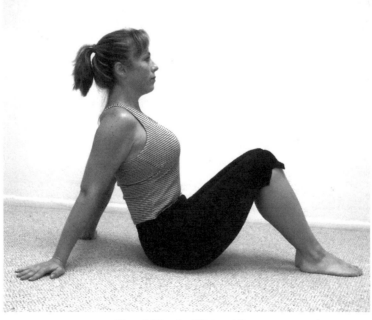

Good Hook-Sit position

Fantastic Feet!

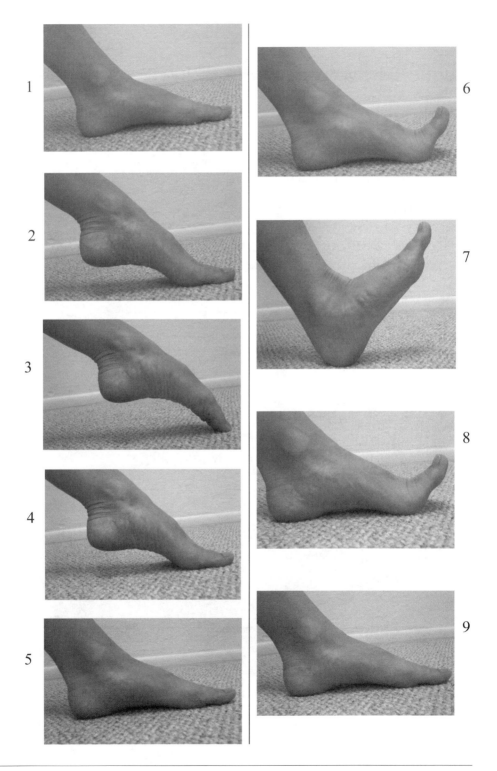

Seated Footwork Exercises

Chair Exercises

If it is difficult for you to get up and down off the floor for the Hook-Sit or L-Sit position, all of the Fantastic Feet exercises can be done seated in a chair. Maintain good posture—sitting tall—at the edge of your seat, while executing your foot exercises. To work the toes, prop your foot up on a stool or bench as needed so you can reach your toes and use your hands for assistance.

For all exercises keep the feet and knees pointed straight ahead. Ankles should not roll in or out. Weight stays evenly distributed between the big and little toe. Heels stay hidden behind the rest of the feet when on your tippy toes.

Recommendation: Do the exercises in front of a full-length mirror to watch leg alignment.

Seated Exercise 1 – Toe Lifts

Begin seated with the feet flat. Inhale to lift the toes off the floor (flex just the toes). Exhale to set the toes back down. Repeat 5-8 times. Be sure the balls of the feet remain on the floor. The big and little toes should lift up evenly. Ankles remain still.

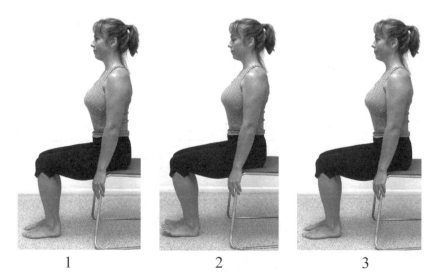

1   2   3

Seated Exercise 2 – Flex the Ankle

Begin seated with the feet flat. Keep the toes relaxed and work the ankle joint. Inhale to flex the ankle, lifting the toes & the ball of the foot off the floor. Exhale to lower the foot back to the starting position. Repeat 5-8 times. Be sure that the feet lift evenly.

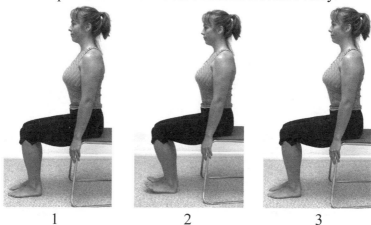

1 2 3

Seated Exercise 3 – Tippy Toes

Begin seated with the feet flat. Inhale to lift the heels as high as possible, so you are standing on your tippy toes. Weight should be evenly distributed between the big & little toes. The ankle should be centered between the knee and toes (not rolled in, or rolled out.) The heels should be hidden behind the feet. Exhale to lower the heels. Repeat 5-8 times.

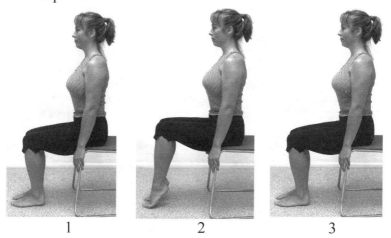

1 2 3

Seated Exercise 4 – Push to Point I

Begin seated with the heels lifted in the tippy-toe position. Keep the heels as high as possible throughout the exercise, inhale to push off the toes to pointed position. Exhale to return to the balls of the feet with the heels lifted high. Repeat this 5-8 times. Finish by lowering the heels to rest.

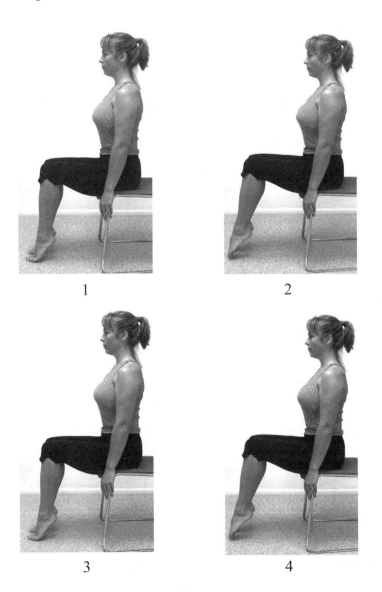

Fantastic Feet!

Seated Exercise 5 – Push to Point II

Begin seated with feet flat. Inhale to lift to the tip toes / inhale to push to point. Exhale to lower the balls of the feet / exhale to lower the heels. Repeat 5-8 times.

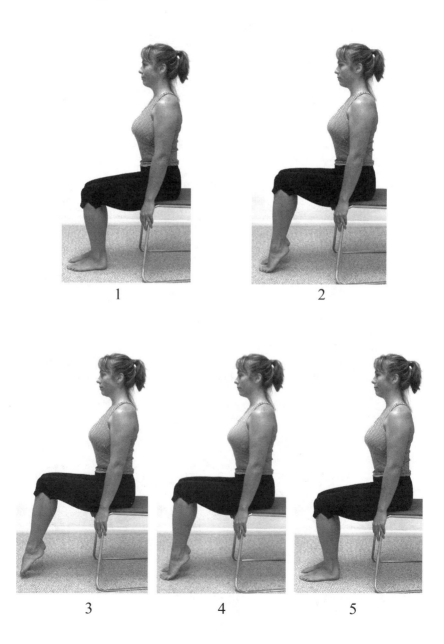

Seated Exercise 6 – Combo: Flex to Point

Begin seated with the feet flat. Articulate through the feet from the toe lifts, to flex the ankle, replace the balls of the feet, then toes to the floor, lift the heels, push to point, roll back down through the feet to the start position. Breathing inhale-inhale, exhale-exhale, inhale-inhale, exhale-exhale. In – toe lifts / in – flex the ankle, ex – balls down / ex – toes down. In – heels lift / in – push to point, ex – balls down / ex – heels down.

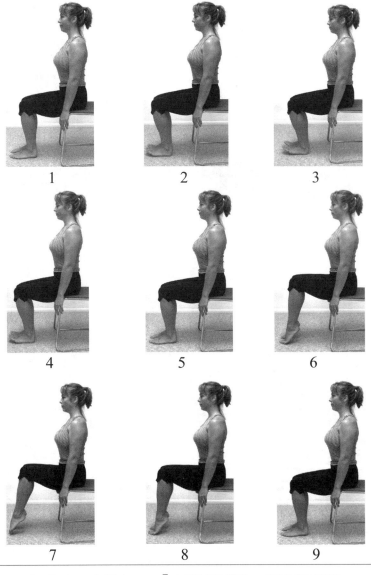

Note for Seated Exercises 5 & 6:

Rather than one long continuous inhale and exhale, breathe with two short inhales followed by two short exhales. The inhale-inhale, exhale-exhale should be crisp. Take in half your breath, then the other half. Exhale part way, then all your air.

You may do these exercises:

a) Both feet at the same time.

b) One foot at a time and alternate legs.

c) Go through several exercises, or the whole series on the right, and then repeat on the left.

Brain Challenge:

Do Exercise 6 with the feet doing different actions at the same time. While the left toes/ankle is flexing, the right heel lifts and toes push to point!

Terrific Toe Series

- Begin seated on the floor, or on the edge of a chair.

- Work with one foot at a time.

- Do all the exercises with one foot, then stand and compare the feeling of lift under the arch and alignment of the feet.

- Repeat the exercises with the other foot.

Knuckles   Reps: 3-5

- Place the fingers under the ball of the foot and lift up.
- Keeping the toes lengthened, wrap the toes around the fingers.
- Use the thumbs to help press the toes down while lifting up under the ball of the foot.
- Try to show all of the knuckles of the foot like you would if you made a fist with your hand.
- Hold for 5-10 seconds, release and repeat 3-5 times.

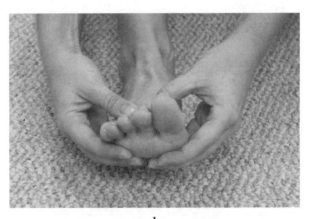

1

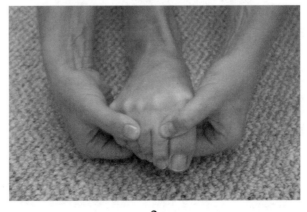

2

Terrific Toe Series

Big Toe   Reps: 3-5

- Place the foot flat on the floor with the toes pointed straight ahead. Keep the toes on the floor throughout the exercise.

- Use one hand to pull the Big Toe towards the midline.

- Hold the toe still and sweep the other 4 toes towards the Big Toe, then away. Be sure the heel stays still.

- Repeat 3-5 times.

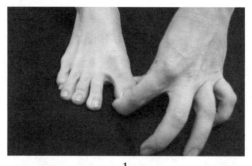

1

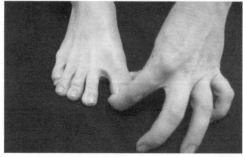

2

3

Little Toe   Reps: 3-5

- Hold the Little Toe and gently pull it away from the body.

- Repeat the above exercise sweeping the other 4 toes away from the Little Toe, then towards it.

- Repeat 3-5 times.

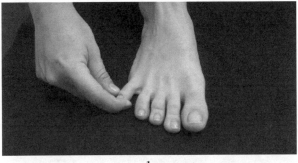

1

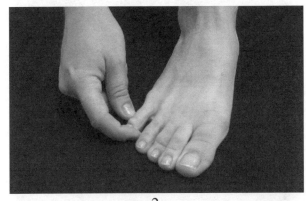

2

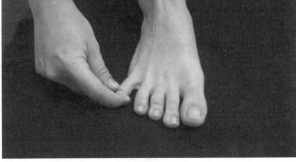

3

Terrific Toe Series

Big & Little   Reps: 3-5

Hold the Big and Little Toe and gently pull them away and apart. Keeping them on the floor, sweep the three toes in the middle to the Big Toe, then to the Little Toe. Repeat 3-5 times.

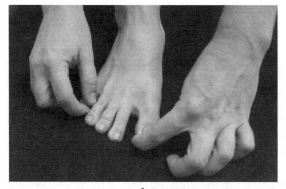
1

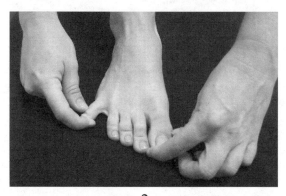
2

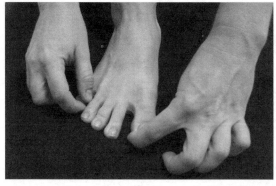
3

Piano Toes   Reps: 3-5 each way

Keep the ball of the foot on the floor and lift the toes up. Hold the toes with the hand and lower one toe at a time back to the floor. Lengthen the toes as they lower. Use the hand to press the toes down if needed and/or hold up the toes that should still be up. Start with the Little Toe and repeat 3-5 times. Then start with the Big Toe and repeat 3-5 times.

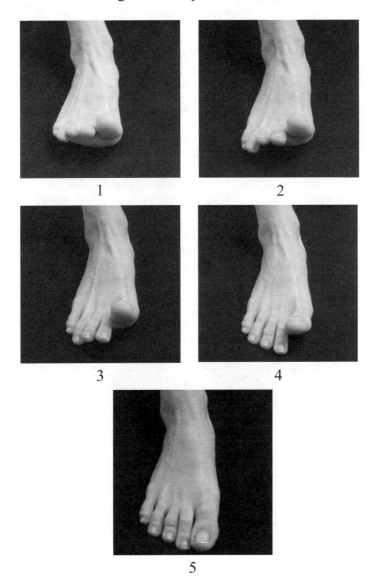

Dome the Foot   Reps: 3-5

Keeping the Big Toe, Little Toe, and Heel firmly planted, lift up under the arch of the foot by contracting the muscles of the arch. Hold for several seconds then release. *This exercise can be done seated or standing.*

Seated Footwork - Dome the Foot

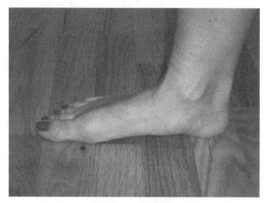

Relaxed Arch

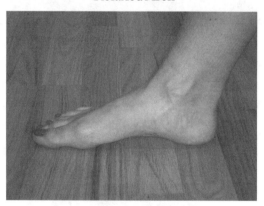

"Doming" Lifted Arch

Notice the angle of the shin in relation to the foot, this is a seated version, and will be easier to start with if you have weak arches or bone displacement probems with your feet.

Progress to doing this in a standing position where you are having to "dome" against the full force of gravity and the muscles of your arch will have to work harder.

Towel Pull & Push   Reps: 3-5

- Lay a towel out flat. Using either one foot at a time, or both, pull the towel towards the body scrunching it up under the arches.

- Pull for 5-10 repetitions.

- Then push the towel back out flat using the toes.

- Push for 5-10 repetitions.

- Repeat this Push & Pull 3-5 times.

- Picking up pencils or marbles also works well for strengthening the feet.

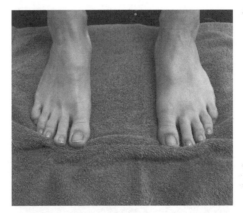

1

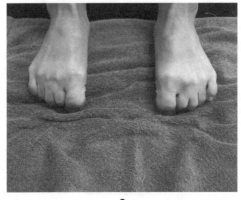

2

Theraband Foot Series

This series of exercises is a fantastic progression from your non-weight bearing exercises to working the toes, feet and ankles in a full-range of motion against resistance.

Originally, these great Theraband foot exercises were created by Deborah Lessen, founder of Greene Street Studio, New York, NY. They were shared with me by my friend and fellow teacher, Dianne Miller.

You will find your weak spots quickly and easily as you work with slow, smooth, control against the tension of the band.

Fantastic Feet!

Theraband Foot Series

The Theraband foot series exercises can be done seated in a chair, or lying on your back. Place the band lengthwise along the entire foot. Hold the ends of the bands with your hands. The tighter you hold the band (closer to your ankle) the more resistance/more difficult the exercise. If necessary begin doing the series without the band. Be sure to maintain good knee/ankle/foot alignment during each of the exercises.

Beginners ~ Do Exercise #1 on the right leg, then switch to do #1 on the left. Continue through the series with #2 right/left . . . etc., Progress to doing #1, 2, & 3 right/left, then #4 & 5.

Intermediate/Advanced ~ Do Exercise #1-5 on the right foot, then switch to do #1-5 on the left foot.

The stronger the Theraband, the more challenging the exercises. Start with a less resistant band. Work to increase repetitions up to 10-12, before progressing to a more resistant band. If you need a real challenge, use 2 bands together for increased resistance and difficulty.

Safety Precaution:
Remove any jewelry and wear socks during these exercises to protect the theraband from breaking. Always check your band before use to insure that it does not have any holes or tears.

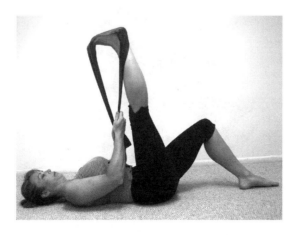

Exercise #1 ~ Toe Curls.

- Flex the foot. (Pull the ankle back towards your shin.)
- Hold the ankle still, and curl just the toes. (Like a monkey, grabbing a branch.)
- Release the toes. Repeat 5 times.

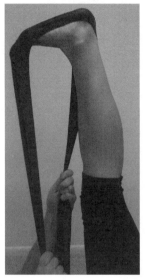
1

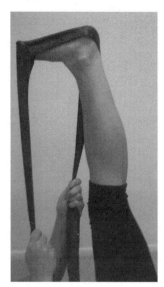
2

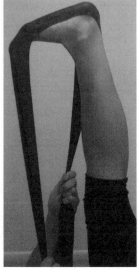
3

Fantastic Feet!

Exercise #2 ~ Point & Flex.

- Begin with the ankle and toes flexed towards your shin.

- Move the ankle first, pointing the foot, then point the toes (like a ballerina on her tip-toes.)

- Release the toes first, then flex the ankle back to the starting position. Repeat 5-10 times.

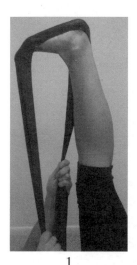 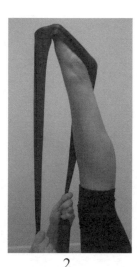 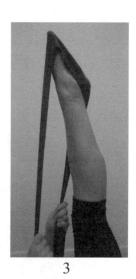

1   2   3

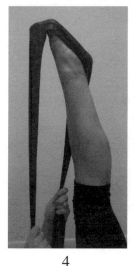 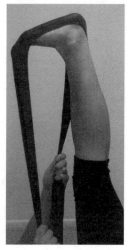

4   5

Exercise #3 ~ Curl & Point.

Starting position as #2 above, only curl the toes first, then point the ankle. Holding the toes curled, flex the ankle back towards the shin, then flex the toes. Repeat 5-10 times.

Exercise shown without theraband for clarity in seeing foot placement.

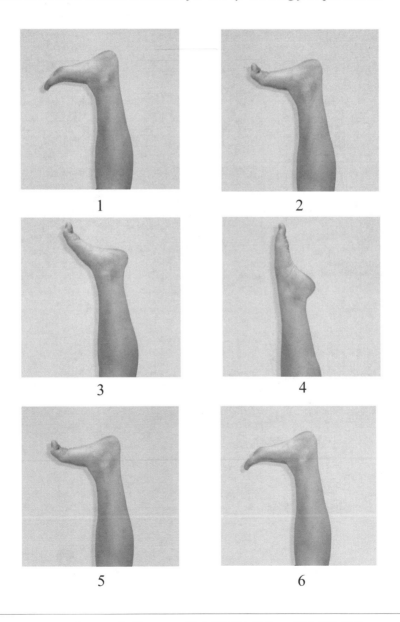

Fantastic Feet!

Exercise #4 ~ Ankle Circles - Away from the body.

Articulate through the toes and ankle while completing big, slow circles of the foot. As the foot moves away from the body, press to the ball of the big toe, and point the big toe first, then one by one from the big toe to the little toe until you are in a good "ballerina point". Hold the point as you pass through the top of your circle, and release the toes from the big toe to the little toe to finish in a strong flexed foot position for a calf stretch. Repeat 5-10 circles in this direction.

Exercise shown without theraband for clarity in seeing foot placement.

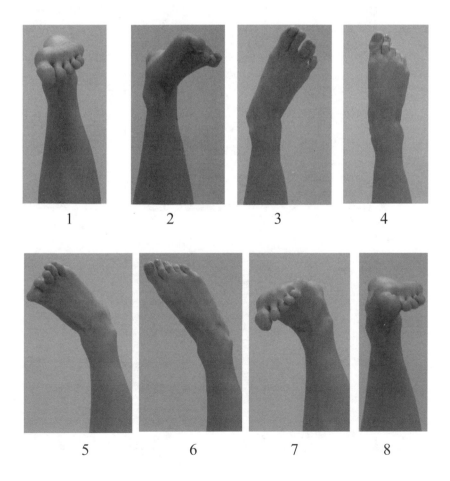

Theraband Foot Series

Exercise #5 ~ Ankle Circles - Towards the body.

Articulate through the toes and ankle while completing big, slow circles of the foot. As the foot moves towards the center of the body, press through the little toe side of the foot—<u>point the little toe first</u>. Then one by one point the toes from the little toe to the big toe until you are in a good "ballerina point". Hold the point as you pass through the top of your circle, and release the toes from the little toe to the big toe to finish in a strong flexed foot position for a calf stretch. Repeat 5-10 circles in this direction.

Exercise shown without theraband for clarity in seeing foot placement.

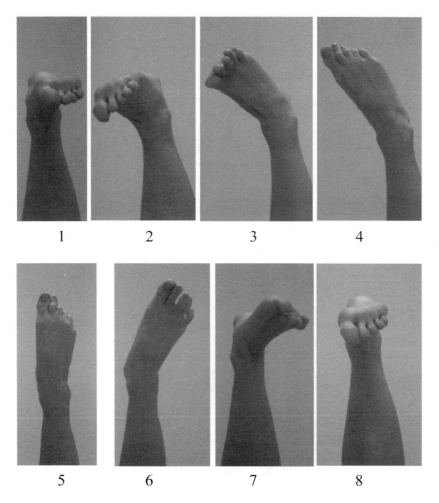

1 2 3 4

5 6 7 8

Standing Footwork Series

The Benefits of Standing Footwork

Standing footwork is beneficial for real life! Once you are aware of proper alignment and posture, practicing good weight bearing on the feet will help to keep your body strong and healthy.

It is much more difficult to change foot, ankle, and leg alignment in a standing position. Our knees take the tork and strain of any improper adjustments. It is much safer and easier to begin making changes in non-weight bearing positions (lying down or seated.) Because of this, work on the Pilates Reformer and Chair along with the fantastic feet exercises can be an excellent way to begin correcting alignment while keeping your joints safe.

Practice your Fantastic Feet exercises in front of a mirror to be sure your alignment is right, you are conscious of your good and bad habits, and are working correctly.

The standing footwork series is also excellent for improving balance and body control. If necessary, start practicing these exercises holding onto a wall or the back of a chair until your balance improves.

Beginners
Begin practicing this series standing flat on the floor.

Intermediate
To increase range of motion, stand on a raised platform or stair—so the heels can lower slightly below floor level.

Advanced Option
For an additional challenge, do the exercises one leg at a time.

Heel Lifts   4-12x

Begin with the feet in a parallel position, toes pointing straight ahead. Legs and feet can be zipped together, or hip width apart to assist with balance. Maintain a good tripod position with the weight even between the big toe, little toe and heel. Abdominals support the body with good tall posture.

Keep the left leg straight, bend the right knee as you lift the right heel off the floor pressing onto the ball of the right foot. Maintain good alignment from the toes to the ankle, knee, and hip. Push from the bottom of the right foot to lower the heel. Repeat 4-12 times on the right, then start left.

Breathing:
   Inhale to lift the heel
   Exhale to lower the heel

Watch that the weight stays even on both legs throughout the exercise. No bobbing and weaving! Be sure the ankle doesn't roll in or out while lifting and lowering the heel.

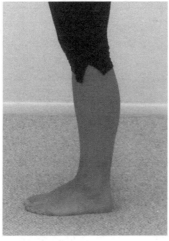

1

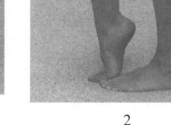

2

Standing Footwork Series

Push to Point   4-12x

- Same starting position as the Standing Heel Lifts.

- Keep the right left leg straight, bend the left knee to press onto the ball of the left foot.

- Keeping the left heel lifted high, push from the bottom of the foot to point the toes.

- Break at the toes to press the ball of the foot back to the floor.

- Roll through the foot to place the heel down.

- Repeat 4-12 times on the left, then start right.

Breathing:
Inhale-heel up, Inhale-point toes
Exhale-to the ball, Exhale-heel down

Maintain good alignment from the toes to the ankle, knee, and hip. Be sure as you point the toes that the bones stay long. Think about pointing to the tips of the toenails (like a ballerina in toe shoes!) Avoid crunching and curling the toes into the floor as you point. Weight should remain even on both legs.

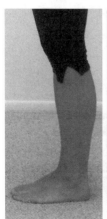
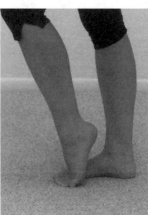
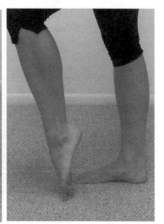

1   2   3

Knee Bends   4-12x

- Same starting position as the Standing Heel Lifts.
- Maintain even weight on the feet. Keep good tall posture.
- Hinge at the hip/knee/and ankle to bend the knees.
- Push from the soles of the feet and engage the gluteal (butt) muscles to straighten the legs.
- Repeat 4-12 times.

Breathing:
   Inhale to bend the knees
   Exhale to straighten

Be sure that the knees don't lock when straightening the legs. It is also very important that the knees line up right over the feet throughout the exercise. Keep the abdominals engaged for support. Avoid tucking the hips, or excessively arching the back. The spine should stay in a neutral position with a normal amount of arch in the low back.

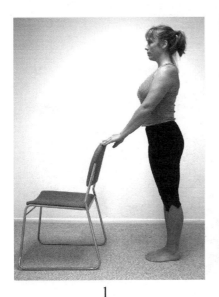

1

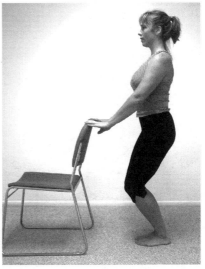

2

Standing Footwork Series

Combo

Do one repetition of the Standing Push to Point on the right, followed by one reptition of the Standing Knee Bend.

Breathing:
  Inhale - heel lift, Inhale - push to point
  Exhale - to the ball, Exhale - lower the heel
  Inhale - bend the knees
  Exhale - straighten the legs

Alternate sides 4-8x

Maintain even weight on the feet, correct ankle/knee/hip alignment, good abdominal support, and tall posture with the shoulders relaxed.

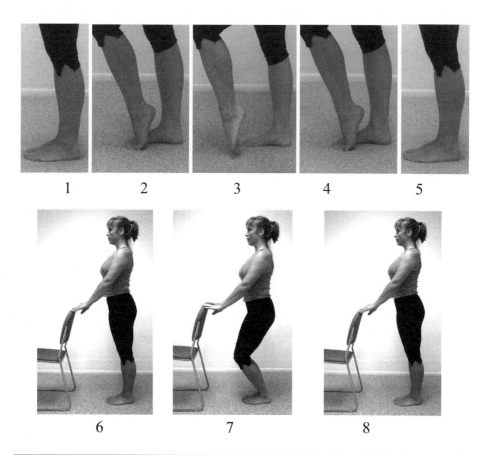

Fantastic Feet!

Lift & Lower   Reps: 5-10

This can be done in a V-position, or parallel. Stand in the selected position. Keep the weight towards the ball of the foot, heel lightly touching the floor. Inhale and rise up on the toes, exhale and lower. Watch leg and ankle alignment both up and down—no wobbles.

> *Watch For:*
> - **In a V-position the heels stay together throughout.**
> - **In parallel, the heels stay hidden from a forward view.**
> - **Maintain balance and control.**
> - **Weight evenly distributed between the big and little toes.**
> - **Avoid wobbles at the ankle.**
> - **Maintain a neutral spine.**

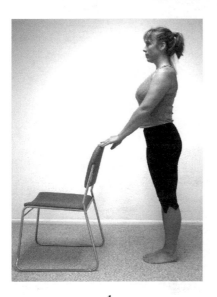

1

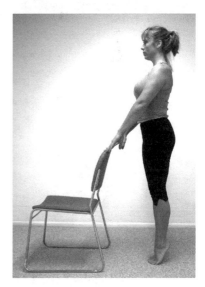

2

Roll Up   Reps: 3-10

This can be done in a V-position, or parallel. Stand in the selected position. Bend the knees, being sure the knees go over the toes. Lift the heels. Straighten the legs keeping the heels lifted. Lower the heels with straight legs. Inhale, Straighten the legs, Exhale, Lower the heels. Watch leg and ankle alignment throughout.

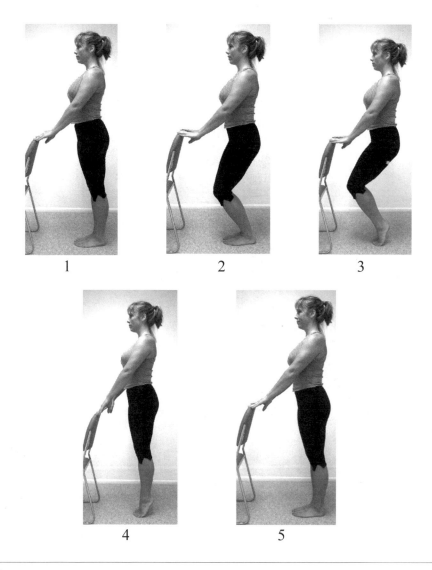

Fantastic Feet!

Roll Down Reps: 3-10

This can be done in a V-position, or parallel. Stand in the selected position. Keeping the legs straight, rise up on the toes, Keep the heels lifted, and bend the knees. Be sure the knees go over the toes for proper alignment. Lower the heels, then straighten the legs. Repeat 3-10 times.

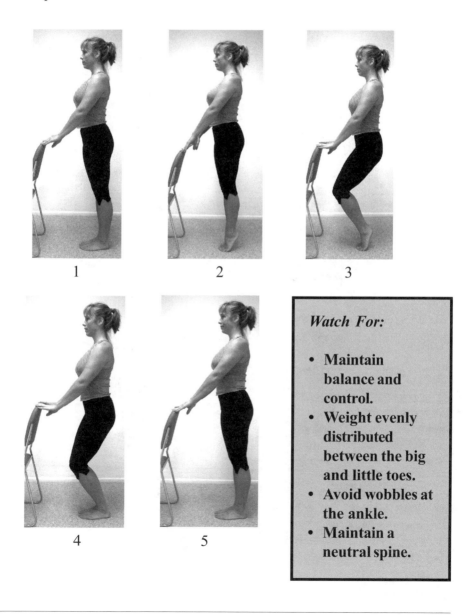

Watch For:

- **Maintain balance and control.**
- **Weight evenly distributed between the big and little toes.**
- **Avoid wobbles at the ankle.**
- **Maintain a neutral spine.**

Standing Footwork Series

Standing Footwork - Rolling Up & Down
(Intermediate Option)

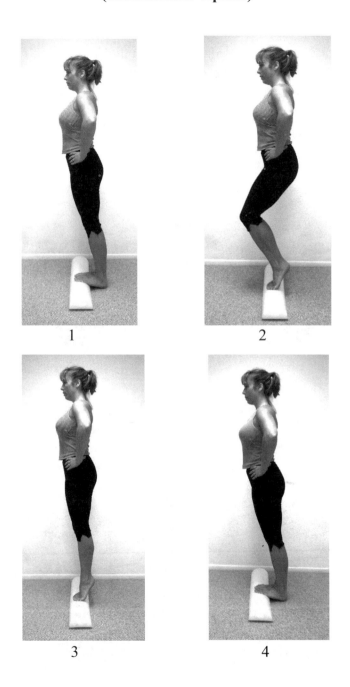

Fantastic Feet!

Prancing in Parallel Reps: 5-10 or more

Prancing can be done slowly to work through the feet, or more quickly to elevate the heart rate. Press to point with the left foot. Return to the ball of the left foot and transition to the right side by rising on the tippy toes. Continue moving, alternating feet. Concentrate on heel—ball-toe as the foot lifts off the floor, and toe ball-heel to return. Work through the feet. The emphasis is UP, a light lifted body.

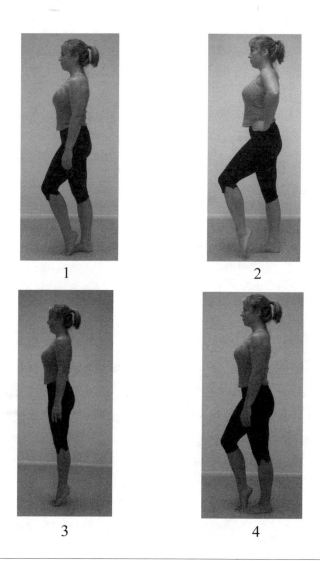

1 2

3 4

Standing Footwork Series

Balance 1 Leg Reps: 1-3 each leg

Balancing exercises work on control and centering. Having good balance is especially important as we age to avoid falls and injury.

All of the standing exercises on two legs are working balance! Having good balance on one leg, will make it that much easier to stay upright on both legs.

To begin stand on one leg and lift the other up slightly—foot by the ankle. Hold as long as possible. Use a wall or barre if needed until balance is more secure. A V-position with the foot on the standing leg will provide a more stable base of support. Practice in a V-position and parallel.

Options for the non-supporting leg:
>Knee Front, Knee Side
>Straight Leg – Front, Side, Back
>Attitude – Front, Side, Back
>More Advanced – balance on the toes

Perception & Awareness Challenge:
Try to balance with your eyes closed. Our eyes play a very important role in providing stability with balance and movement. If you have good balance with your eyes closed it will be even easier with your eyes open!

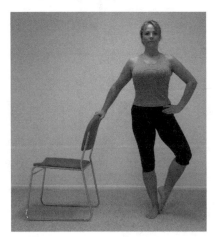
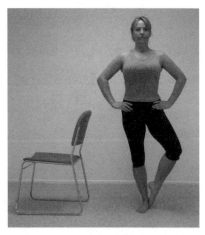

Fantastic Feet!

Quick Reference

L-Sit Exercises
1. Sole Searching, part 1 — 5-10 rep.
2. Sole Searching, part 2 — 3x3 rep.
3. Point & Flex — 5 rep.
4. Toe Curl Combo — 3 Toe Curls/1 Point & Flex - 5 rep.
5. Ankle Circles — 3-5 circles each direction

Hook-Sit Exercises
1. Toe Presses — 3x3 rep.
2. Ankle Hinge — 5 rep.
   a. add toe curls (optional) — 3x3 rep.
   b. Taps (optional) — 20-30 rep.
3. Flex & Point — 3-5 rep.

Chair Exercises
1. Toe Lifts — 5-8 rep.
2. Flex the Ankle — 5-8 rep.
3. Tippy Toes — 5-8 rep.
4. Push to Point I — 5-8 rep.
5. Push to Point II — 5-8 rep.
6. Combo (Flex to Point) — 5-8 rep.

Terrific Toe Series
1. Find the Knuckles — 3-5 rep.
2. Hold the Big Toe — 3-5 rep.
3. Hold the Little Toe — 3-5 rep.
4. Big & Little Toe — 3-5 rep.
5. Piano Toes — 3-5 rep.
6. Dome the Feet — 3-5 rep.
7. Towel Push & Pull — 3-5 rep.

Theraband Foot Series
1. Toe Curls — 3-5 rep.
2. Point & Flex — 5-10 rep.
3. Curl to Point — 5-10 rep.
4. Ankle Circles — 5-10 each direction

Standing Footwork
1. Heel Lifts — 4-12 rep.
2. Push to Point — 4-12 rep.
3. Knee Bends — 4-12 rep.
4. Combo- 2&3 — 4-8 rep.
5. Lift & Lower — 5-10 rep.
6. Rolling Up — 3-10 rep.
7. Rolling Down — 3-10 rep.
8. Prancing in Parallel — 5-10 rep.
9. Balance One leg — 1-3 rep.

> You might find it beneficial to chart your workouts for easy reference.
>
> Please visit:
> www.centerworkspilates.com/logsheet.pdf
> to download this quick reference guide and workout logsheet in pdf printable format.

Standing Footwork Series

Chart your workouts for easy reference.

Download these helpful forms in pdf printable format at:
www.CenterworksPilates.com/logsheet.pdf

Quick Reference Guide

Fantastic Feet Quick Reference Guide

L-Sit Exercises
1. Sole Searching, part 1 — 5-10 rep.
2. Sole Searching, part 2 — 3x3 rep.
3. Point & Flex — 5 rep.
4. Toe Curl Combo — 3 Toe Curls/1 Point & Flex - 5 rep.
5. Ankle Circles — 3-5 circles each direction

Hook-Sit Exercises
1. Toe Presses — 3x3 rep.
2. Ankle Hinge — 5 rep.
   a. add toe curls (optional) — 3x3 rep.
   b. Taps (optional) — 20-30 rep.
3. Flex & Point — 3-5 rep.

Chair Exercises
1. Toe Lifts — 5-8 rep.
2. Flex the Ankle — 5-8 rep.
3. Tippy Toes — 5-8 rep.
4. Push to Point I — 5-8 rep.
5. Push to Point II — 5-8 rep.
6. Combo (Flex to Point) — 5-8 rep.

Terrific Toe Series
1. Find the Knuckles — 3-5 rep.
2. Hold the Big Toe — 3-5 rep.
3. Hold the Little Toe — 3-5 rep.
4. Big & Little Toe — 3-5 rep.
5. Piano Toes — 3-5 rep.
6. Dome the Feet — 3-5 rep.
7. Towel Push & Pull — 3-5 rep.

Theraband Foot Series
1. Toe Curls — 3-5 rep.
2. Point & Flex — 5-10 rep.
3. Curl to Point — 5-10 rep.
4. Ankle Circles — 5-10 each direction

Standing Footwork
1. Heel Lifts — 4-12 rep.
2. Push to Point — 4-12 rep.
3. Knee Bends — 4-12 rep.
4. Combo 2&3 — 4-8 rep.
5. Lift & Lower — 5-10 rep.
6. Rolling Up — 3-10 rep.
7. Rolling Down — 3-10 rep.
8. Prancing in Parallel — 5-10 rep.
9. Balance One leg — 1-3 rep.

Duplication is permitted. Download additional copies at www.CenterworksPilates.com/logsheet.pdf
www.CenterworksPilates.com 1-877-874-7578 or (316) 265-9700
© MMV Aliesa George and Centerworks Pilates®

Workout Logsheet

Fantastic Feet Exercise Training Record

NAME: _____ DATE: _____

- Record the exercises you did in column one.
- Circle the number of reps completed in column three.

My program	Exercise	Goal Reps	My Reps	Notes
L-Sit Exercises				
	Sole Searching part 1	5-10 reps	5 8 10	
	Sole Searching part 2	3x3 reps	2 3 4	
	Point & Flex	5 reps	3 4 5	
	Toe Curl Combo	3 toe curls/1 point & flex - 5 reps	3 4 5	
	Ankle Circles	3-5 circles each direction	3 4 5	
Hook-Sit Exercises				
	Toe Presses	3x3 reps	2 3 4	
	Ankle Hinge	5 reps	3 4 5	
	Toe Curls	3x3 reps	2 3 4	
	Taps	20-30 reps	10 20 30	
	Flex & Point	3-5 reps	3 4 5	
Chair Exercises				
	Toe Lifts	5-8 reps	5 6 7 8	
	Flex the Ankle	5-8 reps	5 6 7 8	
	Tippy Toes	5-8 reps	5 6 7 8	
	Push to Point I	5-8 reps	5 6 7 8	
	Push to Point II	5-8 reps	5 6 7 8	
	Combo (Flex to Point)	5-8 reps	5 6 7 8	
Terrific Toe Series				
	Find the Knuckles	3-5 reps	3 4 5	
	Hold the Big Toe	3-5 reps	3 4 5	
	Hold the Little Toe	3-5 reps	3 4 5	
	Big & Little Toe	3-5 reps	3 4 5	
	Piano Toes	3-5 reps	3 4 5	
	Dome the Feet	3-5 reps	3 4 5	
	Towel Push & Pull	3-5 reps	3 4 5	
Theraband Foot Series				
	Toe Curls	3-5 reps	3 4 5	
	Point & Flex	3-5 reps	3 4 5	
	Curl to Point	3-5 reps	3 4 5	
	Ankle Circles	5-10 each direction	5 8 10	
Standing Footwork				
	Heel Lifts	4-12 reps	4 8 10 12	
	Push to Point	4-12 reps	4 8 10 12	
	Knee Bends	4-12 reps	4 8 10 12	
	Combo 2&3	4-12 reps	4 8 10 12	
	Lift & Lower	4-12 reps	4 8 10 12	
	Rolling Up	4-12 reps	4 8 10 12	
	Rolling Down	4-12 reps	4 8 10 12	
	Prancing in Parallel	4-12 reps	4 8 10 12	
	Balancing One Leg	4-12 reps	4 8 10 12	

Duplication is permitted. Download additional copies at www.CenterworksPilates.com/logsheet.pdf
www.CenterworksPilates.com 1-877-874-7578 or (316) 265-9700
© MMV Aliesa George and Centerworks Pilates®

Foot Reflexology and Massage

In the practice of Oriental Medicine different parts of the feet are associated with different organ systems. Tender spots on your feet, could be an indication of poor health in other parts of your body.

So aside from the benefits of stronger and more flexible arches, ankles and toes through the practice of your Fantastic Feet exercises, taking the time for a good foot massage can keep your whole body feeling better.

Use the following Reflexology Chart as a reference to a help give your feet a treat. Pay attention to any tender areas. By practicing your Fantastic Feet exercises, and finishing with a foot massage, you should quickly begin to notice improvements.

Fantastic Feet!

REFLEXOLOGY CHARTS

This chart serves as an instant introduction to the popular massage practice of reflexology. The history o reflexology dates back to ancient China, 4000 or more years ago. The technique is natural, does not require drugs and can be applied to both, hands and feet. The soles of the feet and palms of the hands divide into sections that mirror the different body organs. Massaging these areas can stimulate and strengthen the associated internal organs and promote wellbeing. The procedure brings relaxation and ease to the whole body. It assists in restoring and maintaining a healthy balance of body and mind. Even the simplest massaging of the fingertips dan be very pleasant. Revitalize your body and mind by applying reflexology massages in your home or place of work.

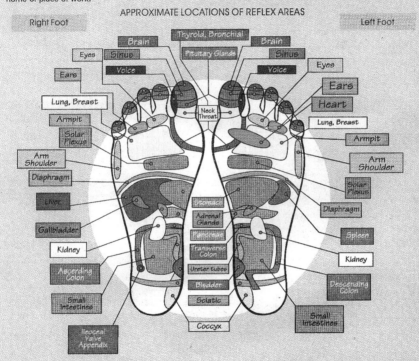

APPROXIMATE LOCATIONS OF REFLEX AREAS

RELAXING THE HANDS	HOLDING WITH EVEN PRESSURE	THE FINGERS	RELAXING THE FINGERS

Hold both hands loosely, facing downward. Gently shake then for 1 minute.	Wrap the fingers around tose. Use the thumb to press them slightly backwards.	For those areas the thumb cannot reach. Bend fingers on first joint, push tops forward.	Hold each finger in turn firmly and pull with gentle force.
KNEADING ACTION	**THUMB IS IMPORTANT**	**USE LEVERAGE**	**ROTATING ACTION**
Form a fist and use it to knead plams and soles. Alternate hands.	Slightly bend thumb on first joint. Repeatedly pust tip forward by straightening joint.	Make sure that thumb and fingers are always opposite each other for good leverage.	Hold limb, rotate gently around ankle or wrist in alternating directions.

www.CenterworksPilates.com ▪ 1-877-874-7578 or (316) 265-9700

© MMV Aliesa George and Centerworks® Pilates Institute

About the Author

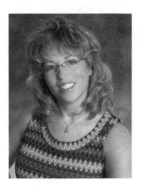

Founder and President of Centerworks® Pilates, Aliesa George is committed to helping people develop their belief in unlimited potential and positive change, by increasing awareness through mind, body, and movement.

Aliesa has been sharing her experience and expertise for over 25 years as a Pilates teacher, presenter, and wellness professional. She has written, and continues to write, many educational books and articles relating to Pilates, posture, movement, and whole-body health.

Aliesa has a degree in Modern Dance from Texas Christian University, is a Gold-Certified as a Pilates Teacher through the Pilates Method Alliance, ACE Certified Personal Trainer and Group Exercise Leader, and is certified as a teacher of Bigu Qigong for weight-loss, weight-management by the International Institute of Chinese Medicine.

Her Personal Mission:

To inspire others to think, learn, and grow—by lighting the path and teaching the personal steps needed to achieve success for revelation and evolution into a healthier, happier life.

Centerworks® Pilates Institute

For information on hosting a workshop or seminar and to order additional educational tools available from Centerworks, please contact:
Centerworks® Pilates Institute
P.O. Box 3526
Wichita, KS 67201-3526
Phone/Fax 1-877-874-7578 or phone (316) 265-9700
www.CenterworksPilates.com
email: info@CenterworksPilates.com

References

Muscles Testing and Function (4th edition)
Florence Peterson Kendall, Elizabeth Kendall McCreary, Patricia Geise Provance
Williams and Wilkins (1993)
428 E. Preston Street
   Baltimore, Maryland 21202
   ISBN # 0-683-04576-8

Taking Root To Fly
Irene Dowd (1998)
   14 East 4th Street #606
   New York, New York 10012
   ISBN # 0-9645805-0-0

Dance Technique and Injury Prevention
Justin Howse
   Routledge (2000)
   29 West 35th Street
   New York, New York 10001
   ISBN # 0-87830-104-6

Anatomy of Movement
Blandine Calais-Germain
   Eastland Press, Inc. (1993)
   P.O. Box 12689
   Seattle, Washington 98111
   ISBN # 0-939616-17-3

Therapeutic Exercises - Foundations and Techniques (3rd edition)
Carolyn Kisner, Lynn Allen Colby
   F.A. Davis Co. (1996)
   1915 Arch Street
   Philadelphia, Pennsylvania 19013
   ISBN # 0-8036-0038-0

Recommended Resources

Visit www.CenterworksPilates.com

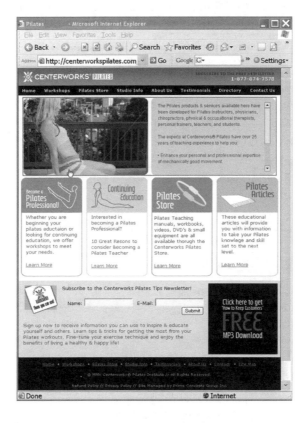

For additional copies of this book visit:
www.Foot-Care-Help.com

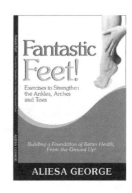

Recommended Resources

The Fundamental Training Series: Posture Principles for Health

If you've been looking for an easy-to-use system for posture evaluation here it is! This must have posture workbook and video will provide you with the tools you need to quickly identify poor posture habits and help clients change.

Included is a 12-point checklist for perfect standing posture, seated posture pointers, a series of questions to help you and your students quickly become aware of posture habits, teaching tips and more. This information is great client "homework." A good place to start when developing workout programs to promote efficient movement and good health.

  √ **Enhance Posture**
  √ **Improve Awareness**
  √ **Get Results!**

Posture Principles for Health Video & Study Guide (60 Pages)
Order # PP-VHS - VHS Format $79
Order # PP-DVD - DVD Format $79

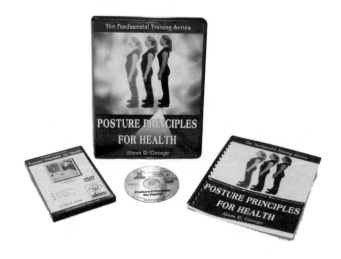

Get the Entire Set of Centerworks® Pilates Teacher-Training Manuals

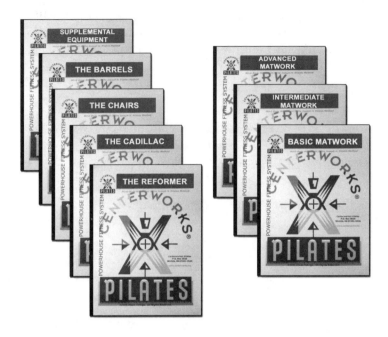

This series of eight Pilates Training Manuals is one of the most comprehensive Pilates resources available on the market.

Hundreds of pictures, detailed exercise descriptions, repetitions, breathing, safety guidelines, and modifications.

All the information you need to know to safely and effectively teach the Pilates repertoire. A great addition to your education!

Get the Complete Set of 8 Pilates Teacher-Training "How-to" Manuals.

Basic Matwork   *Intermediate Matwork*
Advanced Matwork   *Supplemental Equipment*
The Reformer   *The Cadillac*
The Chairs   *The Barrels*

Order #TT-ALLBK Teacher Training Set *(printed manual)* **$225**
Order #TT-ALLEb Teacher Training Set *(PDF download)* **$177**

Recommended Resources

Centerworks Pilates Teacher-Training Manuals

This series of Pilates Training Manuals is one of the most comprehensive Pilates references available on the market. Hundreds of pictures, detailed exercise descriptions, repetitions, breathing, safety guidelines, and modifications. All the information you need to know to safely and effectively teach the Pilates repertoire. *(All 8.5x11)* A great addition to your education!

You'll learn:

- √ Step -by-step details for proper execution of over 200 exercises
- √ Cautions for clients with special problems
- √ Appropriate repetitions & breath patterns for each exercise.
- √ Equipment set-up & safety tips. Guidelines for modifications and variations.
- √ Important points to pay attention to when teaching exercises

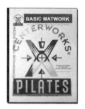

Basic Matwork 80 pages - 22 exercises - 141 photos.
A detailed plan to teach and progress students through the beginner Pilates Matwork. Learn the first 22 exercises, and how to sequence a workout as taught in a "traditional" Pilates Mat class. Also included: an outlined teaching plan to introduce & teach the basics.
Order #TT-BM01 $25 printed manual *or*
#TT-ebBM $17 PDF download

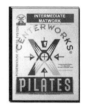

Intermediate Matwork 68 pages - 12 intermediate exercises (31 exercises total) - 151 photos.
Progress students into the intermediate Pilates Matwork. By following this systematic approach, your students can increase their strength & flexibility building on the basics.
Order #TT-IM02 $25 printed manual *or*
#TT-ebIM $17 PDF download

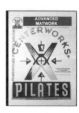

Advanced Matwork 56 pages - 23 exercises - 130 photos
The complete repertoire of Advanced Matwork. Guidelines for layering the exercises into an intermediate workout. This manual contains only the advanced Matwork exercises. Best suited for teachers & experienced Pilates students who are ready to work at this level.
Order #TT-AM03 $25 printed manual *or*
#TT-ebAM $17 PDF download

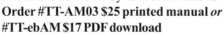

www.CenterworksPilates.com ▪ 1-877-874-7578 or (316) 265-9700
© MMV Aliesa George and Centerworks® Pilates Institute

Supplemental Exercises 57 pages - 35 exercises - 128 photos
A great addition to your "bag of tricks" for teaching Matwork classes. The exercises in this manual utilize, the wall, hand weights, and the Pilates Magic Circle. This manual goes great with the Intermediate Mat book.
Order #TT-SP04 $15 printed manual *or*
#TT-EbSP $10 PDF download

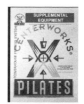

The Reformer 117 pages - 58 exercises - 147 photos
Step-by-step guidelines to learn & teach the beginner and intermediate Pilates Reformer. Lots of pictures, precautions for working with special problems, equipment set-up, repetitions, and safety.
Order #TT-RF05 $40 printed manual *or*
#TT-EbRF $32 PDF download

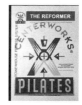

The Cadillac 113 pages - 60 exercises - 353 photos
All of the Pilates equipment exercises assist in lengthening & strengthening for a total body workout. An "ideal" workout includes Reformer, Matwork, and additional exercises as needed with the other "supplemental" pieces of equipment. Continue developing strength, stability, & flexibility with the Pilates Cadillac.
Order #TT-CA06 $40 printed manual *or*
#TT-EbCA $32 PDF download

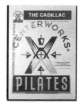

The Chair 74 pages 46 exercises - 108 photos
Contains both Electric Chair & Wunda chair exercises. The chair exercises are great for strengthening hips & knees. Before the Stairmaster, there was Joseph H. Pilates and the Wunda Chair! An amazing piece of equipment that can stand alone for a great total body exercise program.
Order #TT-CH07 $40 printed manual *or*
#TT-EbCH $32 PDF download

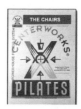

The Barrels 100 pages - 37 exercises - 243 photos
A great encyclopedia of Ladder Barrel, Spine Corrector, and Small Barrel exercises. The barrels are a wonderful way to increase spine mobility and improve posture. Add this to your Pilates library!
Order #TT-BA08 $40 printed manual *or*
#TT-EbBA $32 PDF download

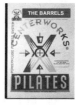

Recommended Resources

The Centerworks® Pilates Audio Workout Programs

These Pilates Audio books have been designed to challenge your mind and body—and are offered at all levels, so you can pick the most appropriate place to start, and will always have options to pick up the pace, or slow things down and do some fine-tuning.

Each Audio workout will cover traditional Pilates Matwork exercises—no two tapes will be exactly alike. By finding different ways to challenge you to think about what you're doing, and learning ways to make each exercise easier or more challenging. These Centerworks Pilates Audio Books are currently available in MP3 as an online download, and on CD. Put your Pilates workouts on your IPod for a supplement to your Cardio training. Great for travel too!

Basic Pilates – Flowing Fun: The First 15 Matwork Exercises
Designed for the newer Pilates student, this audio workout focuses on getting strong with the Basics. This class is slower paced for the less experienced students to concentrate on finding the right stuff with the first fifteen Pilates Mat exercises. Gain strength, flexibility and confidence with this Basic Pilates Mat class. 37:30 min audio
Order #FLO1 Audio CD $12 *or* #MP3-FLO1 Audio MP3 $10
BEST DEAL! Order #AUD-CD-FLO1 Audio CD & MP3 combo $17

**Beginner-Intermediate Pilates – Gearing Up: Matwork with Flow
23 Exercises**
This audio is a good, solid Pilates Mat class. Designed for beginner and intermediate level students, to think, work, and move. Pick up the pace, add eight new exercises to your basic workout program, and increase your endurance with this class. Develop your proficiency and fine-tune your technique. If you never learned another exercise…this class will keep you focused and fit. 41:10 min. audio
Order #FLO2 Audio CD $12 *or* #MP3-FLO2 Audio MP3 $10
BEST DEAL! Order #AUD-CD-FLO2 Audio CD & MP3 combo $17

**Intermediate Pilates Matwork – Flowing Fitness Challenge:
37 Exercises**
A vigorous & challenging class for all experienced Pilates enthusiasts. Plenty of cues to tweak your technique, while you move through thirty-seven intermediate level Pilates Matwork exercises. Trim your rim, get in touch with your center, and tone your whole entire body with this great audio workout. 1 hr. 12 min. audio
Order #FLO3 Audio CD $12 *or* #MP3-FLO3 Audio MP3 $10
BEST DEAL! Order #AUD-CD-FLO3 Audio CD & MP3 combo $17

Order Your Audio Workouts at www.CenterworksPilates.com Today!

Pilates Magic Circle

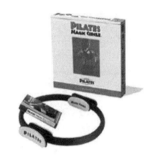

A great tool for increasing the resistance and challenge of your Pilates workout. Also great for stretching! Improve your muscle tone and endurance with the Pilates Magic Circle from Stamina®. This kit includes the effective Magic Circle and a motivational video. The Pilates Magic Circle was created by Joseph Pilates to be a versatile exercise aide you can use anywhere.

It provides resistance for faster, more targeted toning, improving muscle strength throughout the body...especially in problem areas.

Pilates Magic Circle and Video. Order #SE-MC01 $30

Pilates' Return to Life Through Contrology

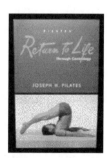

Return to Life is the original Pilates exercise book written by the creator and visionary of the Pilates method of exercise, Joseph H. Pilates. This book review the conceptual basis and philosophy of the Pilates method or "Contrology" and the original Matwork exercises Mr. Pilates taught in the studio on 8th Avenue and 55th Street in New York City. The model featured in this book is Mr. Pilates himself at the age of 60.

This book was originally released in 1945. Reprinted in 2003, with great quality photos.

A "must-have" book for your Pilates library. Order #JHPBK1 $14.95

Therabands

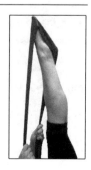

Resistant Exercise Bands for Muscle Strengthening. Assistance for correct technique, and great for travel. Package of 2 bands $10.

Beginner~Yellow/Red Order #SE-YR02 $10
Intermediate~Green/Blue Order #SE-GB03 $10

Recommended Resources

Stress Reduction Course
52 Weeks to a Happier Stress-Free Life

Do you find your self nearing the end of your rope? Are your nerves frazzled? Are the pressures from work and the demands of your family starting to take their toll on your health?

In the fast-paced world we live in today, there are so many factors that add to our stress levels. Work/or lack of it, spouse/children/parents, finances, school, time, politics, world issues, pollution, war, technology, traffic . . .

Just because we are used to having stress in our lives, it doesn't lessen the negative and harmful effects these stressors can have on our health. The world around us may be in turmoil but there is much we can do to create peace within.

Aliesa George has been sharing the secrets of health and wellness for over 25 years, teaching traditional physical exercise programs, weight loss/weight management courses, and Pilates—movement for health. By encouraging the development of the mind-body connection and increasing awareness for positive lifestyle changes, she has had the privilege of watching people make amazing changes that have dramatically improved their quality of life.

You can now get the benefit of Aliesa George's stress-management tips and tricks that she has shared with private clients, workshops and presentations, in her 52-week internet course:
Tips & Tricks for a Stress-Free Life.

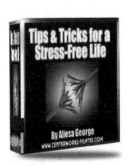

Get the information you need. Learn at your own pace. Improve the quality of your life and enjoy better health with this effective 52-week course: ***Tips & Tricks for a Stress-Free Life.***

Visit www.StressManagementHelp.com to get started on your stress reduction course today!

Fantastic Feet!

Suspended Motion Bronze Pilates Sculpture
by artist Donna Cooper

This Pilates-inspired artwork will look great in your home or studio! This work was commissioned by Centerworks® Pilates to honor the first Annual PMA Pilates Day. A portion of the proceeds fromeach piece will be donated to the Pilates Method Alliance.

Don't miss your chance to show your Pilates Enthusiasm, and help support the PMA!

PILATES ART - Limited Edition, Bronze Sculpture

Details:
- Bronze Sculpture 14" h x 10" w
- Black marble base
- with beveled edge 12" x 4" x 1"
- Total dimensions 14" x 18" x 10"
- Approximate weight 17 lbs.

Special - Limited Offer
Only $895 Save $100 (Reg. price $995)
Hurry & order - This special price is available for a limited time.

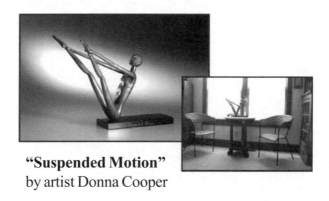

"Suspended Motion"
by artist Donna Cooper

www.CenterworksPilates.com ▪ 1-877-874-7578 or (316) 265-9700

© MMV Aliesa George and Centerworks® Pilates Institute

Recommended Resources

For More Information About Pilates

Centerworks® Pilates Institute
For information on teacher training, hosting a workshop or seminar and to order additional educational tools available from Centerworks, please contact:
    Centerworks® Pilates Institute
    P.O. Box 3526
    Wichita, KS 67201-3526
    Phone/Fax 1-877-874-7578 or phone (316) 265-9700
    www.CenterworksPilates.com
    email: info@CenterworksPilates.com

Centerworks® Pilates Institute is a Corporate and Training Member of the Pilates Method Alliance.

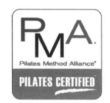

Aliesa R. George is a PMA Gold-Certified Pilates Professional.

The Pilates Method Alliance
If you are interested in furthering the work of Joseph & Clara Pilates as a business, teacher or fitness enthusiast, please consider joining the Pilates Method Alliance. You may also use the PMA to help you locate Pilates teachers and studios in your local area. Your support is appreciated!
    Contact the PMA at:
    The Pilates Method Alliance
    P.O. Box 370906, Miami, FL 33137-0906.
    Phone 866-573-4945 Fax 305-573-4461
    www.pilatesmethodalliance.org
    email: info@pilatesmethodalliance.org

How To Order

Name_____

Company_____

Address_____

City_____ State____ Zip_____

In case we have questions about your order:

Office_____ Home_____

Cell_____ Fax_____

E-Mail_____

For shipments to an address other than your own, fill in below:

Name_____

Address _____

City_____ State____ Zip_____

Phone_____

INTERNET: www.CenterworksPilates.com
PHONE: 1-877-874-7578 or (316) 265-9700
FAX: 1-877-874-7578
MAIL: Centerworks® Pilates Institute
         P.O. Box 3526
         Wichita, KS 67201-3526 USA

Method of Payment:

Check or Money Order payable to: Centerworks Pilates (No cash or COD's please.)
We accept: Visa   M/C   AMEX
Card Number:

_ _ _ _ _ _ _ _ _ _ _ _ _ _ _ _

Card Expires _____/____

Signature_____

Item Number	Description	Quantity	Price Each	Total

SHIPPING CHART
Economy Small Package Shipping U.S. Priority Mail

IF YOUR ORDER TOTALS	PLEASE ADD
$50.00 and under	$ 6.50

Fed-Ex	Standard	2nd-Day
$25.00 and under	$ 8.00	$ 19.00
$25.01-$ 50.00	$ 9.00	$ 20.00
$50.01-$100.00	$ 11.00	$ 21.00
$100.01-$200.00	$ 15.00	$ 26.00
$200.01-$300.00	$ 19.00	$ 41.00
$301.00-$400.00	$ 24.00	$ 57.00
$400.01-$500.01	$ 34.00	$ 77.00
$500.01 and over	$ 49.00	$104.00

Shipping Charges Subject to Change

Sub-Total _____

7.3% sales tax KS residents _____

(see chart) Shipping _____

Add 10% for Alaska, Hawaii and Canada
Add 20% for Foreign and Overseas

Sub-Total _____

TOTAL _____

30-day - 100% money back guarantee on items returned in resalable condition.